PRANAYAM
KHEL KHEL MEIN

PRANAYAM
KHEL KHEL MEIN

PRAMILA IYER

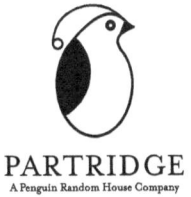

PARTRIDGE
A Penguin Random House Company

To order additional copies of this book, contact
Partridge India
000 800 10062 62
orders.india@partridgepublishing.com

www.partridgepublishing.com/india

Dear Readers!

No pain no gain…so goes the adage! Such a prophetic statement for me, for I became a Yoga Teacher because of my back ache!

I attributed my back ache to my professional life (life of a couched-potato working as a stenographer) and I almost accepted the pain as a part of my life. The pain sometimes was so unbearable that I was put on pain-killers and ignorant that I was at that period of my life that I thought I was cured by those magic pills! I did not know then, that 'relief' was not necessarily a 'cure'. Slowly I got hooked on to the pain killers as I had two boisterous boys to look after. A day came when even pain-killers were not giving me relief, and I was screaming with pain. I was barely 33, and my doctor, to my great relief said that my bones were o.k., but the muscles needed some toning-up and some exercise. I thank the doctor,(and also the pain,!) which took me to one of the best yoga teachers in Pune.

To cut my story short, yoga changed my life totally! I started reading many books on yoga and its philosophy, and by the age of 37, I was teaching and preaching yoga left, right and centre. The yoga aphorisms seeped into my being so much that I knew I had started on a joyous new journey towards the Creator. Apart from the physical aspects – the postures - which is just a tip of the iceberg, yoga philosophy viz. yama, niyama, pranayama, pratyahara, dharana, dhyana and samadhi – the 8 limbs of yoga, brings about a totally different approach towards life itself. It is very unfortunate that people think of "yoga" as some postures and deep breathing exercises.

I am deeply indebted to all my yoga teachers from different schools of thought. In one of the classes I attended, they did not teach pranayam till your body was properly trained by doing various asanas and made more supple. I was very keen on learning pranayamas from that particular yoga school, but I had to wait for quite sometime till they felt I was ready. I was disappointed and this disappointment lead to another yoga school (I had learnt yoga from four different schools of yoga and thus enriched myself greatly) and in course of time, I trained myself to be Yoga Teacher, and I was teaching it totally free of cost, with missionary zeal. I had the good fortune of working in a hospital, remand home, ITI etc, and each and every student became my teacher in a way, helping me to use different props, to suit the individual needs. Every time I was teaching yoga, it was like a very deep communion with my Creator. Instead of blindly teaching what I had learnt, I relied on my intuition and deep connection to God and deeper commitment to my students. As this was neither accepted nor appreciated by the organization under whose banner I was working then, I bid farewell and started my own style of teaching never forgetting to quote and explain the yoga aphorisms. The only question which troubled me was, "Why do some yoga schools/teachers have so much reservation/ apprehension about teaching pranayama to a beginner?" Then I asked myself; "who taught me to breathe when I entered the world?" My mother? My doctor? The nurses? None of them... I could breathe on my own. Yes I was born with the knowledge of how to keep myself alive for which I had only to breathe! I learnt it without being taught!

I went down in my memory lane. Probing into my own childhood, I got more and more insight. I knew Simha Mudra even as a young girl of 9 or 10, for, did I not frighten my little brother by opening my mouth wide, hanging my tongue out, squinting my eyes, and roaring like a lion ? Hurray ! I knew Simha Mudra without being taught! I was doing pranayama naturally...when my nose was blocked, did I not (I still do) close one nostril and trrrr blow from the other? If this action is called as kapalbhati in yogic terminology, who taught me kapalbhathi? And I was doing Pranayam naturally....This being the case, why do some yoga teachers insist on learning asanas first, before learning pranayams? Some of them even frighten the students by saying that doing pranayams without a guru can be dangerous. We are all breathing...correctly... or...incorrectly. (that is another question.) But, we do breathe...don't we? Do we fear? Certainly not...may be we fear "what if I don't..(breathe) (which means death)and not what if I(breathe).... While I do appreciate the care and concern of my well-meaning teachers, I still feel, the fear is totally unwarranted. Yoga and pranamaya is very scientific. In any form of science; there are do's and don'ts, which is more as a precaution than to frighten students. Like, kumbhak:(retention of breath).. whether internal or external, needs a guide, a teacher. Otherwise, people can safely practice many of the pranayamas and also, all the pranayamas given in this book-let. In fact, those of you who wish to teach the breathing techniques, please practice them for a few weeks, till you are confident about them.

My main purpose, as I said in the beginning of the booklet, is to teach Pranayam, naturally. I bow my head in reverence to the little ones for their enthusiasm, energy, open-mindedness and most of all, fearlessness in entering into something new. They are born to learn…to experiment and experience --. without inhibition or hesitation. I salute all the children of the world and this booklet is an offering to the limitless powerhouse called "children". CATCH THEM YOUNG, DEAR PARENTS AND TEACHERS AND GOOD-HEALTH AND GOOD-LUCK TO EVERY ONE!.

I also welcome the YOUNG AT HEART to join these children to bring back your own childhood and experience new thrill, new joy and new life through these pranayamas…and I promise you that..

PRANAYAM...KHEL KHEL MEIN (the joy of "breathing techniques")

Most of the children like company. They enjoy and learn faster in group activities. As such, before we start our "**pranayama khel khel mein,**" form a small group of 20 to 30 children. It would be a great idea to have their mother/father/guardian to attend the introductory lecture where you can brief them about your session.

Here I have divided all the pranayams in different scenes/settings. To make it interesting, I have tried to depict each pranayam through pictures on the opposite page. According to books on yoga, mudras and kriyas are different from pranayams. Since, our main purpose is to enjoy better-health, we side-step all the technical jargons. To learn more about mudras and kriyas, please contact yoga teachers personally.

Children love to hear stories. And if the person is adept at story-telling, there will be good rapport between the teacher and her/his students. Story telling is a great art. Bodily gestures, voice modulation, tone, etc, play a great role is delivering the techniques and the message effectively.. Children tend to get bored easily, if there is no fun in whatever they are learning.

(SOME SUGGESTIONS TO THE TEACHERS TO TEACH THE PRANAYAMAS IN A STORY FORM)

TEACHER:

Dear Children,

Shall we go on picnic to a big forest with many tigers, lions monkeys?

THE CHILDREN:

Yes miss, we are very eager to see all the animals.

THE TEACHER;

How shall we go,? by bus or train? (she pretends to be thinking of some choices of transportation and discusses about air pollution/noise pollution etc. and suggests using of bicycles whenever/wherever possible to avoid polluting air.

THE TEACHER; Hey, we shall go on our cycles? Is it not a great idea?

(Let them share their views on pollution /noise created by vehicles etc related to traveling by mechanized vehicles.)

THE TEACHER: o.k. let us go on our bicycles. Oh! Because we did not use them for some time, we need to pump air into them.

(Before teaching this breathing exercise, the teachers can practice the same in their houses with a real cycle-pump to get the feeling of pumping action, so that it becomes easy for them to teach.)

CYCLE PUMP

Method: Standing posture...make fists ...inhale and raise your hands...exhale and bring down the hands..

Repeat the action for 3 to 5 minutes:

Teacher: That was great! Shall we go now?

Children: yes, madam!

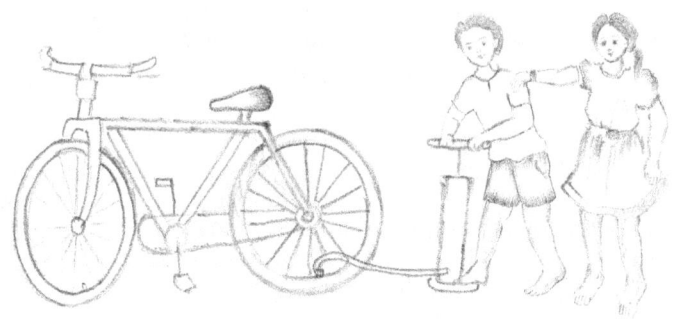

Lesson 2

DOG BREATHING

Children love animals, (well...most of the children do) especially the young ones. It would be a great idea to bring a pet dog (the friendly one, of course!) or still better, a pup. -Before teaching them "dog-breathing", let them observe how the dog/puppy breathes, how it gently shakes its whole body with the tongue hanging out... ask them to become doggies, and they learn without your teaching!

Benefits: Oxygen intake is increased many folds and this gives them tremendous energy...no need for artificial supplement ...gives the benefit of physical exercise without tiring them in the process.

Duration:15 to 20 seconds ...rest for 1 minute... Repeat. 3 to 4 times.

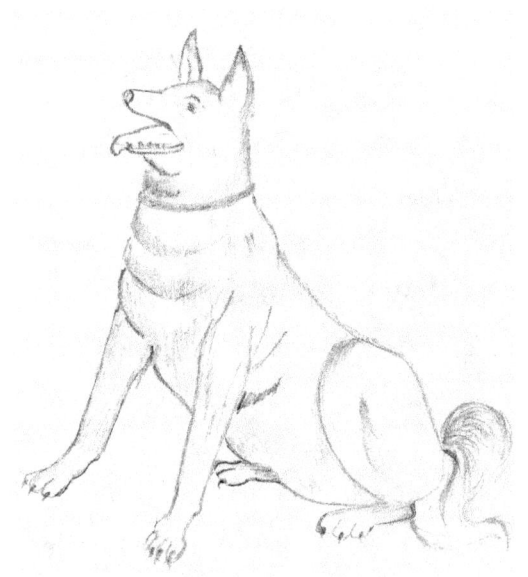

SIMHA MUDRA

(Creating a Scene)

Please, don't get me wrong…..,<creating a scene> literally means that.. creating a "jungle like" atmosphere. If circumstances permit, take the children to a park or an open space with some trees… if that is not possible, (in case if you are teaching them in the class room/or your house etc) try to have a few cut-outs of animals.) Alternatively, children can also wear masks of animals. If all of them have lion-mask, nothing like that! A pride(literally and figuratively, too) of lions with their full-throated roars will soar through the sky!

Method.

Make them sit in vajrasana (sitting on legs folded at the knees) Palms are kept on the floor, fingers spread-out like fans. Let them gently raise themselves supporting their weight on the palms... eyes are fixed in between the eye-brows. ..tongue hangs out and every body will make a "roaring sound"

Benefits: throat gets cleared...eye muscles get gentle massage...very effective for asthma patients and for throat problems.

Let them roar according to their full capacity... Repetitions: 3 or 4 times, with few minutes rest in between.

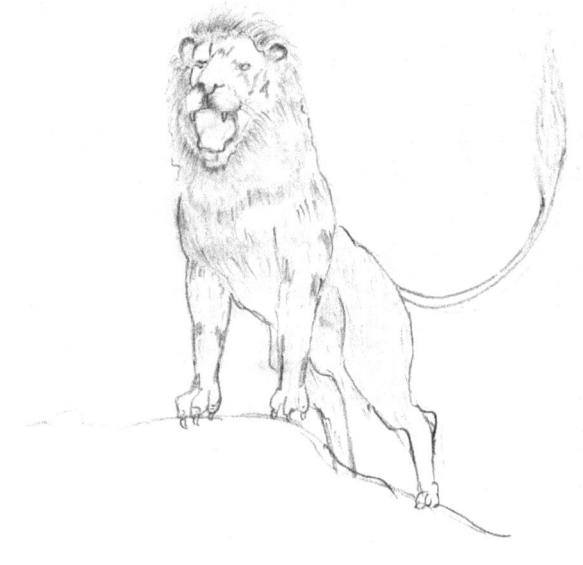

Lesson 4

TORTOISE BREATHING

Is there a baby-pool in your school? Great ! If not, you can use a plastic tub filled with water and if possible float a rubber or plastic tortoise in it..(just to create an ambience.. that is all) Please, use only tortoises, as otherwise, the children will get confused.

The technique: let the children sit comfortably. Inhaling they raise their head up and exhaling they bring their chin to their chest

Benefits: good exercise for the neck and upper part of the chest- more ventilation in the neck region- relaxes the neck muscles.

Stretching and relaxing of the neck muscles activates the thyroid glands thus helping them in their growth process.

Repetition; 10/20 inhalations and exhalations.

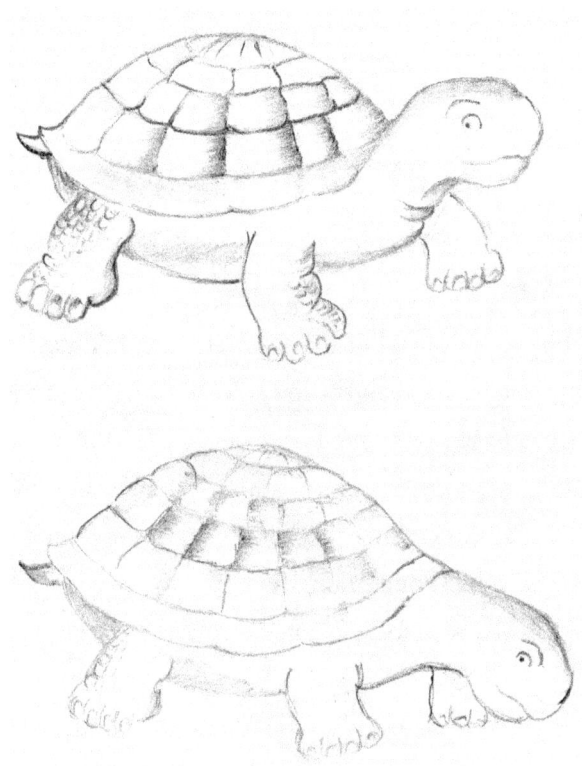

RABBIT BREATHING

The technique:- Let the children sit in vajrasana. The tongue is kept between the lower lip and the lower teeth-. mouth is partially opened and hence breathing is done through the nose as well as the mouth. Very gentle yet active breathing as their bodies also move in synch with their breathing.(For a dramatic effect, you may give them some carrots, which they can eat after the session.)

Benefits: It is like a general tonic- all-round benefit.

Duration 10/20seconds...rest for few minutes.., repeat 3 to 4 times.

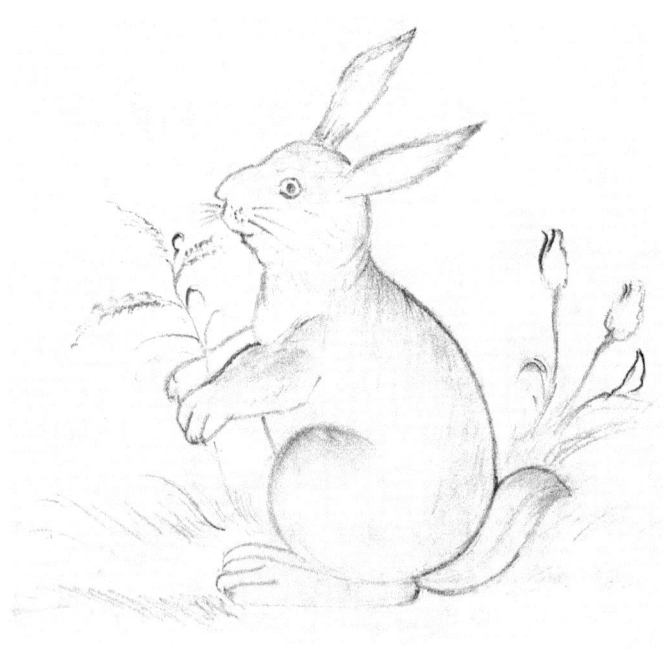

BUMBLE BEE BREATHING (BHRAMARI)

The technique: Let the children sit on the floor, if possible in padmasana. Inhaling deeply, they exhale making a humming -like sound by vibrating the vocal chords.. The sound resembles that of humming of a bee..

Benefits: Nose/throat gets cleared

Duration: as long as it is comfortable to them – Repetitions 3 to 4 times

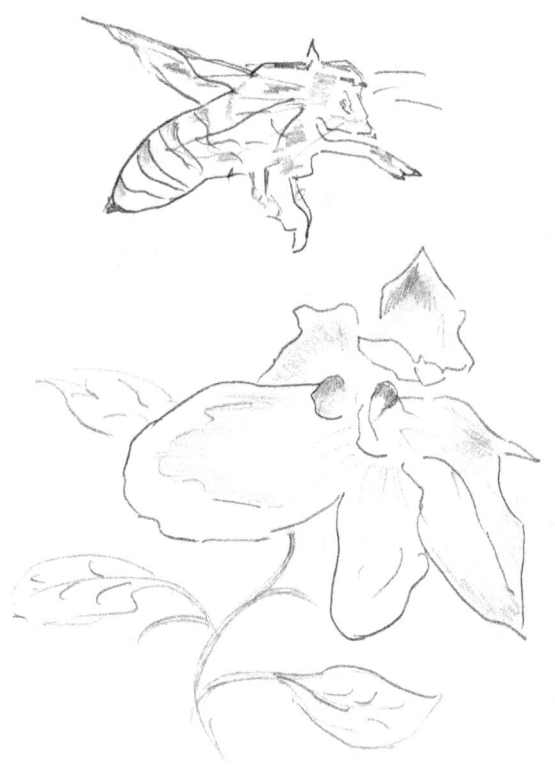

CHUK CHUK GADI -
the good old steam engines.

Dear teacher:

Home work is necessary for a teacher as well, for she/he has to prepare the subject thoroughly before teaching the same to the students. As it is always better to practice before we teach, try this exercise at home. I am sure, sometime during your childhood you have played this game. I am only refining it a little from the standpoint of "breathing exercise" instead of just another "game".

Technique: open one of your hands..four fingers stay together, while the thumb is moved away from the rest of the fingers...the angle of thumb and the pointer finger is kept near the lips (thumb goes below the chin...pointer almost touches the nose) and short blows of air is thrown at the angle. If you get a heavy metallic sound, yes you got it alright! Even if it is not so heavy, still it is perfectly alright

Duration: just enjoy a long ride by the country side!

The story moves further thus......

Teacher:

Oh that was a long ride is it not? What does smoke do to our dress? Yes! They become dirty. Shall we get them cleaned?

A suggestion: The plastic baby-pool or a tub filled with water will make it very interesting for children to learn this pranayama, as they always like to play in water.

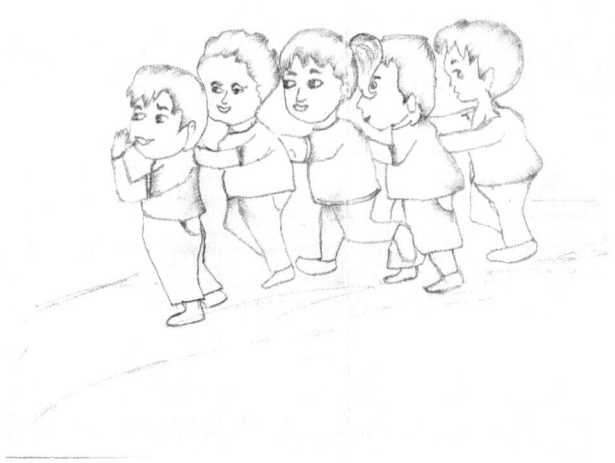

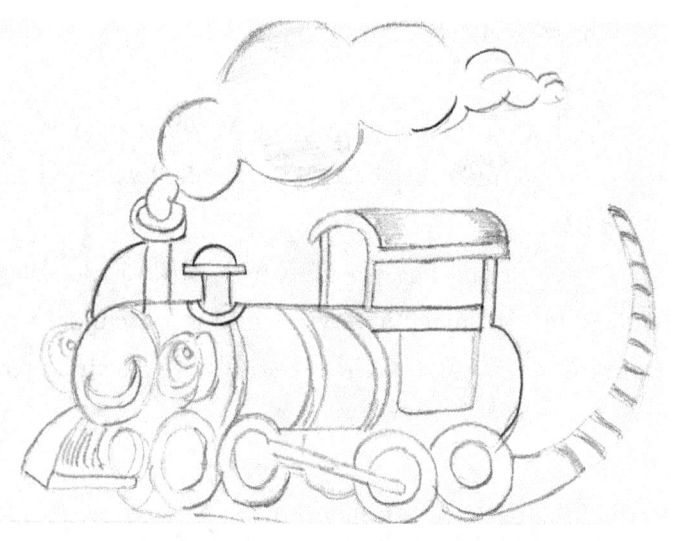

DHOBI KA GHAT
(the washermans' water-hole)

Keep some towels ready. Take one of them, (wet it if weather permits it) raise it in the air, and bang it on the floor. Because we are learning breathing exercises while washing clothes also, emphasis is on synchronizing inhalation and exhalation with the banging of the cloth. Inhale and lift...exhale and bang!

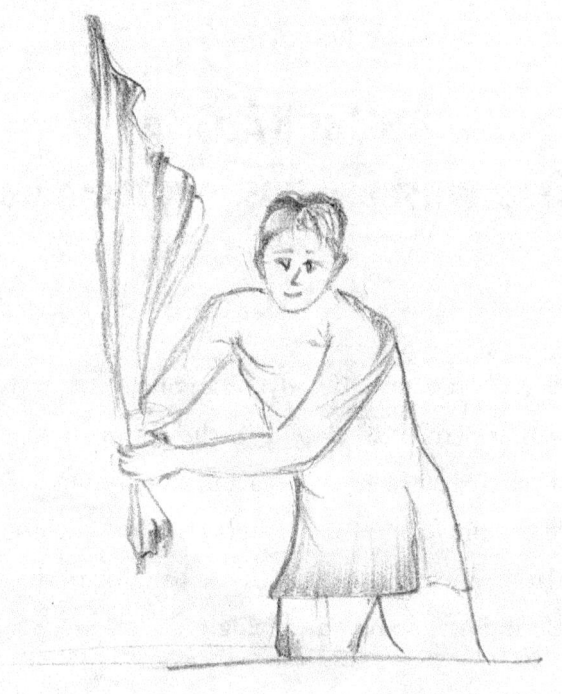

THE WINGED WONDERS ..

To the teachers: Create some story about any bird of your choice and include some information about them.

Many children spread their hands and make flying actions. In fact, I learnt this from them, and I am teaching this back to them with a little modification. The flying action can be a another pranayam khel khel mein when we synchronize their breathing with the action. As the hands which are held parallel to the floor rise up, let them inhale...and exhale as they bring them down.

To the teacher; For the next pranayama, some brief information can be given about village life, their hard work, etc. We can also include the farmers because of whom we get our supply of our grains, pulses etc. Talk about their relatives in villages so that it becomes inter-active.

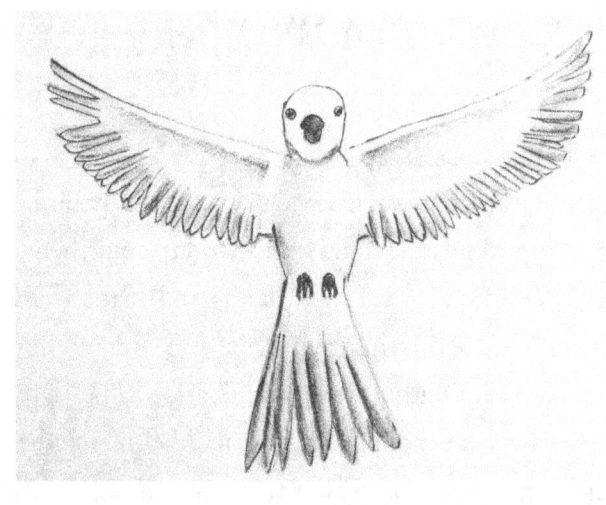

POUNDING RICE/ MASALA etc

Is there any need to teach how to do it? And that is pranayam khel khel mein..!

Well, just for your information, let the children make pounding action by inhaling and rising their hands, and exhaling and bringing the hands back to the original position.

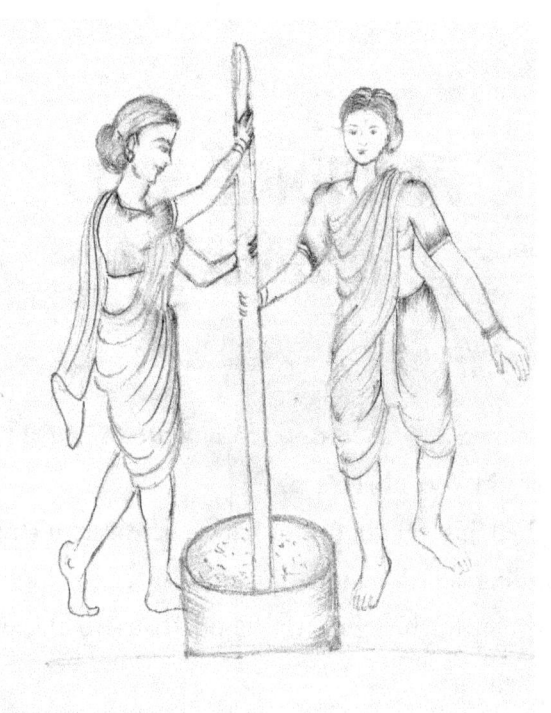

HAPPY BIRTHDAY TO ALL!

Children are always extremely exited about their birthdays. The birth-day boy/girl is a v.i.p. on that day and he is surrounded by all his friends and relatives. The beautifully decorated cake is kept on the table, and he blows out the lighted candle signifying a landmark is his life.

In this technique, the lighted candles will be kept 1 or 2 meters away (cakes and other goodies which go with the birthday party depends entirely on the teacher, but having lighted candles is a must)

Let them inhale deeply (the stomach bulges a little, as they do it) and they completely exhale and extinguish the candle! (The distance between the child and the candle can be adjusted according to their age)

Birthdays are incomplete without games! Keep few balloons ready and let each child get an opportunity to blow at least one balloon (keep a few balloons extra, in case!…)Blowing air into balloons by itself is a great way to increase our lung capacity.

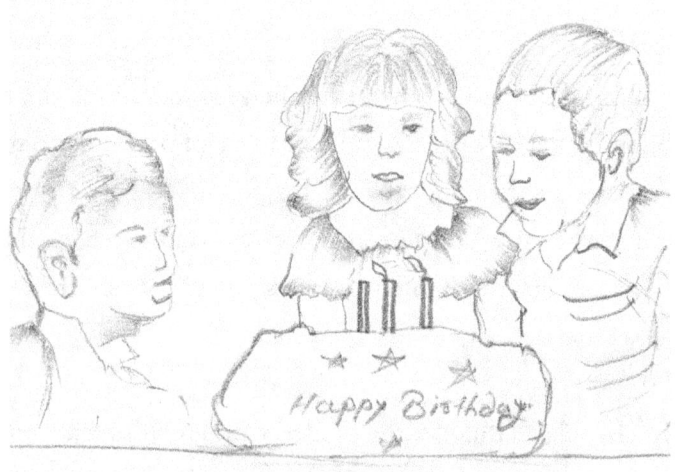

ICECREAM PRANAYAMA!

The most favourite eatable of the young and the old is undoubtedly the ice-cream.

Ask them to do the following pranayams without telling them the title. Ask them to share the experience after doing it. Every body will tell you about the chillness felt in the mouth and the throat. A light-hearted explanation can be given as to how to keep cool during summer/ while traveling through deserts or where water is not easily available. But, at the same time, benefits of having good amount of water should also be stressed upon.

a. Sithali: the tongue is folded like a beak, and air is sucked in through the mouth….ask them to share their experience..99% of the children will tell you

how cool they all felt…yes..as the name suggests –
sithali – is a cooling pranayam.

I am sure, dear teachers, by now you know what item
is involved in this pranayama…yes..the most sought after
eatable for the young and the old for most of the people
of the world …:Ice cream!

b.   Sitkari: tongue is kept on the upper palate behind
the teeth….through the open mouth, air is sucked
in and gulped down….

c.   Sadanti: teeth are clenched.. and air is sucked
through the mouth and gulped down

Sithali, sitkari and sadanti, are cooling pranayams.
Very beneficial during summer days.

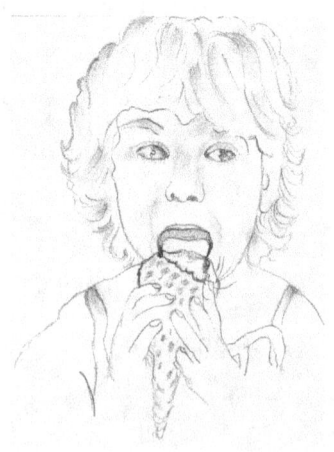

EAT WITH YOUR NOSE!

(The above title can be used when your students are above the age of 10...for children below that age group avoid using 'eat with your nose' for in their innocence, they take every thing literally, but never the less, let them enjoy eating with their nose. For this pranayam, keep some fresh fragrant flowers (no artificial perfumes, please!). Let them inhale deeply and exhale through their mouth making a 'haaaa' sound

As body and mind are intrinsically related, doing pranayama regularly will bring out many latent talents.

Be it blowing off the lighted candle or inflating a balloon, the breathing becomes deep and exhalation deeper. Winding up this session with cakes and goodies where everybody celebrates their birth-day brings such joy not only for the children but also to the teachers as well.

And thus ends our Pranayam Khel khel mein (playful-pranayams) bringing great happiness and good health to these 'bundle of joy', 'apple of parents' eyes..(use every possible endearments in all the languages you know, for, dear readers, for me my whole life in revolved around children and children alone! I experience closeness to God with children. I love them, as I love God!

Sai Ram!

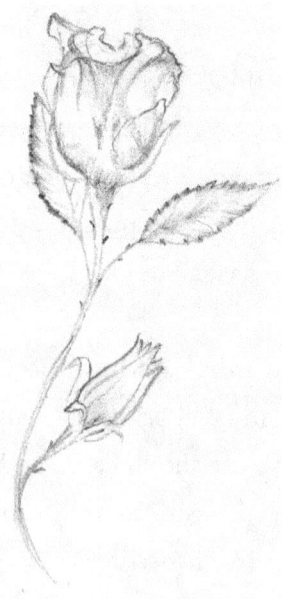

Message for the teachers

DEAR TEACHER Congratulations and felicitations from all of us from Divine Help Centre, a registered charitable trust, working in social, educational and spiritual field. Educating the masses is our motto and mission. Learning a technique and then teaching it will reinforce your own learning. Sharing of knowledge, and not storing it, will expand it more and more. The world needs you...the children need you and we owe our success in spreading this <Pranayam khel khel mein> to YOU AND YOU ALONE. Thank you all, my unknown pals, may we meet sometime during this lifetime. Adieu! God Bless All

Just the beginning…..for a life time of good health, joy and peace!

Breathing exercises gives tremendous energy to our whole system. It is like earning money. You earn money and you also set aside some amount in a bank for future use. Is it not? Though it is not possible to "store" our breath, for future use, nevertheless, by practicing yoga nidra after pranayama is recommended so that energy is not leaked or squandered away.

YOGA NIDRA (YOGIC SLEEP)

Nature's greatest gift is good-sleep. And some people are a little-less gifted when it comes to getting good sleep. People with sleep disorder will not mind doing anything to get some good-sleep. Because, it is mainly during our sleep our body's rejuvenating system works its maximum so that the next day you can do your work efficiently. In fact, denying a person his sleep is practiced also as a torture method, by the police and by the military on the prisoners of war to extract information/confession etc. In fact, I heard a story about how some scientists were given anti-sleep injections for a week, which made them forget even their own names. Such is the power of sleep or the lack of it.

Yoga nidra-the yogic sleep – is an amazing technique for rejuvenating the whole body and mind.

The technique: Let the children lie flat on a carpet. Legs are slightly and comfortably spread apart. The hands are kept away from the body, with the palms facing upwards. Eyes are gently closed. Head is comfortably kept either at the center or on one side. The emphasis is on individual comfort. A soft and sweet voice giving instruction to relax the body from feet to head (starting with toes upwards) brings a total relaxation.

Suggestion: Tape your own voice giving the necessary instruction....replay it....note down how you feel about your own voice … make few changes to create a very soft soothing sweet instruction...almost like a lullaby... so that the listeners are drifted away into deep peace and tranquility..

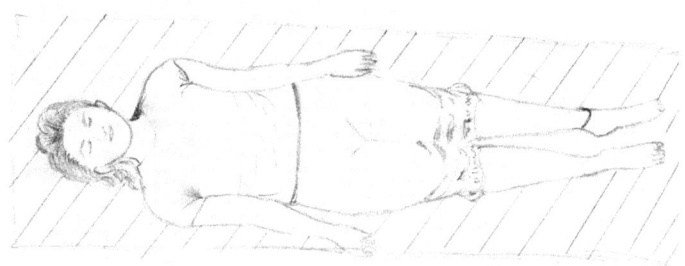

YOGA NIDRA ...the procedure.

Start from the left small-toe move them a little...tense them a little and relax them...then the feet..and thus each and every part of the body is tensed and relaxed. This deep relaxation activates their sub-conscious mind and the benefits of this relaxation is tremendous; Towards the end of the session, while the children are still deep in their total relaxation, you can add a few positive sentences also.. for example during exams or just before them, try with the following suggestions;

1. I have good memory.
2. I am confident about myself.
3. I enjoy studying
4. I am lovable

Depending on the age group, you can include some affirmative sentences. If you are handling tough teen-agers with unwanted addictions, like drugs, alcohol or smoking, please use this opportunity to do the greatest service to humanity. Only in English grammar, two negatives make one positive. But in yoga nidra, two negatives do not make a positive. E.g. do not give suggestion. "I am not addicted to tobacco" ...instead suggest;

1. "I am free from my addiction of tobacco" or better still... "I have clean habits"
2. I have good relationship with my family and friends
3. I am always in good company

Every teacher knows the miracle of encouraging words...use it liberally ...

Schedule: Choose any one or maximum two of the pranayams...always end the session with yoga nidra...

Suggestion: best done in the morning. There should be a gap of at least 1 or 2 hours if they are doing pranayams after breakfast. The best option is...let them have their morning tea/coffee/milk empty their bowels and then get into the session. If you prefer to teach them in the evening, there should be gap of minimum 3 to 4 hours after lunch. Unlike adults, children digest food better and faster. And as such, the time gap between meals and pranayama need not be very rigid as in the case of adults.

Hope you enjoy "Pranayam khel khelmein" with your students, friends and relatives.

God Bless!.